HOLISM, HOMOEOPATI
and the HEREA

This is an excellent review, understandable by the man in the street, of what I would call 'spiritual medicine'. It gives very readable descriptions of the subtle bodies, karma, reincarnation, guidance from higher realms, and many other important subjects, relevant to all of us, and particularly to those practicing medicine in a truly holistic manner.

There is no book that I have come across that describes all these subjects in one connected book in such a straightforward, simple manner. I hope this book gets the wide readership it deserves.

Julian Jessel-Kenyon
Co-Director, Centre for the Study of
Complementary Medicine.
Director, The Dove Healing Trust

HOLISM, HOMOEOPATHY, HEALING AND THE HEREAFTER

To Olive,
with lots of love
Barrie

BARRIE ANSON DHoM, MRadA, DHD.

Wessex Aquarian
— Publications —

Published in the UK

1992

Published by
Wessex Aquarian, P.O. Box. 1059,
Sturminster Newton,
Dorset DT10 1YA.

Cover illustration by Peter Greenhill

ISBN 0-9516963-1-9

Typeset in Century 13/14pt by Scriptmate Editions

Printed on re-tree economy paper by
Booksprint,
31 Clerkenwell Close, London EC1

Acknowledgements

I would like to acknowledge, with gratitude, the many helpful comments from different friends who have assisted in the preparation of this book. In particular I would like to thank Heather Agnew, Keith & Willow Ellis, Pete and Gilly Greenhill, Angela Howe, John Lloyd, Mary Robinson and Josephine Sellers for their special contributions.

The quotation on pages 85 to 87 is from *Sunrise*, published by The White Eagle Publishing Trust of Liss, Hampshire, U.K., and is used with kind permission.

About the Author

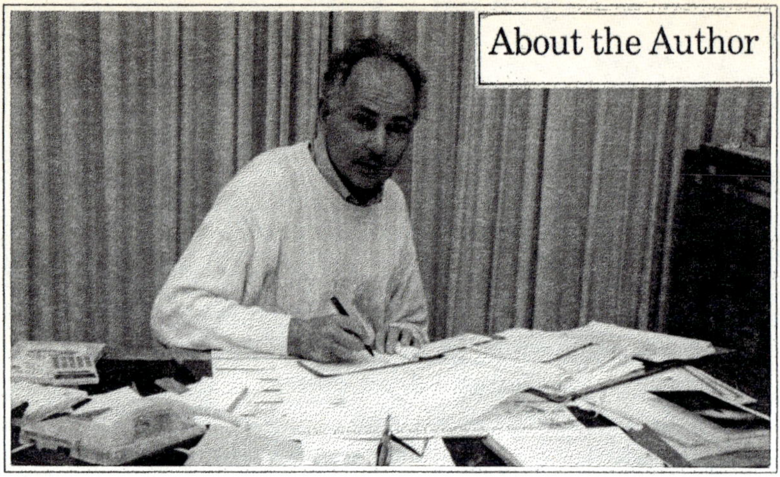

Barrie Anson was born in 1938, brought up in the New Forest area and educated at Brockenhurst School.

He completed a 'thoroughly undistinguished' two years of compulsory National Service in the Army, a year of which was served in Hongkong.

He then began a marketing career in the Pharmaceutical Industry. Initially working in London his career then continued in the Far East where he was based in Bangkok, Thailand. After some years in Thailand as Marketing Manager for an American drug manufacturer he was later posted to Lagos, Nigeria.

Following a personal crisis he opted out of 'big business' to live in Athens, Greece. After a series of adventures there, and much international travel, he lived briefly in France where his interest in spiritual matters began to emerge.

Returning to England in the late 1970s, the author worked in the health food trade, later training in Homoeopathy, Radionics and Dietary Therapy. He has been in practice for the last 13 years and lives in Poole, Dorset with his wife Veronica (a Counsellor and Healer) and two cats.

This book is dedicated to W.E.
and all workers for the Light.

'Deliver us from these human forms and reclothe us in light among the stars'

Nosairi Prayer.

'A little while, a moment of rest upon the wind, and another woman shall bear me'

Kahlil Gibran in The Prophet

Foreword

by Dr. Marianne E. Harling. BA, BM, BCh, FFHom

Holistic healing should take into account everything about the patient—body, mind and spirit, and this includes his attitude to death; for death is a part of life, the other side of the coin, the start of a great adventure.

'In my end is my beginning'

(T.S. Eliot—East Coker.)

People have always feared death, the unknown, and one of the purposes of religious systems was to help control this fear—or sometimes to capitalise upon it! In today's materialistic and scientific age an increasing number of people grow up without a spiritual tradition. Such religion as they may have been taught in childhood was thrown out with the fairy tales (another rich source of spiritual nourishment). However, people are soul and spirit, as well as body and mind, and as they grow older, expecially if health fails, they begin to wonder about the meaning of life and death. Death is a taboo subject in the modern world, so these questions are suppressed into the unconscious, where they generate fear which in turn leads to further disharmony and ill-health.

In former times, as in Egypt, Epidauros, and the

medieval monasteries, and still in primitive societies wherever they exist, priest-physicians or shamans were concerned with the physical, mental and spiritual welfare of their patients. Today the two professions, priest and doctor, have been sharply segregated. The doctor treats his patient's body (or if he is a psychiatrist, mind), but stops short of discussing spiritual matters, especially death, which is regarded as a medical failure, and therefore unmentionable. The priest may be called in, but often not until the patient is dying, or even dead. (The relatives will not send for the priest sooner, in case the sight of a clergyman 'frightens the patient to death').

Holistic medicine, such as homoeopathy, which proceeds at a more relaxed tempo than orthodox medicine, should provide an ideal opportunity for exploring the spiritual issues. Unfortunately fear and embarrassment often prevent the subject from being raised, and the patient is faced with a bright goal of endless physical health, with the shadow of death conspicuous by its absence. Unformulated questions are neither asked nor answered. Experience has shown that when these anxieties can be expressed, the result is a deeper bond between therapist and patient which leads to a more complete healing.

Such cases are described in this book, which has been written by a practising homoeopath and healer, to let light into a dark corner. First a comparison between orthodoxy and holistic medicine shows the suppressive nature of the former—nevertheless he believes that co-operation between the two methods is preferable to polarisation. Next follows a clear and concise description of homoeopathy, its origins and philosophy, and how it works to promote self healing.

Diet, with particular reference to vegetarianism, correct breathing and other aspects of healthy living are then discussed.

In the second part of the book the writer tells us about his own experiences, and the concepts which have helped him, and later his patients to realise their spiritual dimension. These subjects include reincarnation, karma, free will, angels, the subtle bodies and the experiences of people who have almost died but have returned to life. They form part of the Ancient Wisdom teachings which are to be found in the scriptures of all religions, and in the collective unconscious of the human race. Not everyone will accept his views, some people feeling more comfortable with the belief they already hold. This will in no way dismay the author, whose aim is not to convert, but to provide for those who are unsure, afraid or perplexed, a starting-point from which each can make his own individual journey. There are many ways to climb a mountain.

This book is lucid, simple and a pleasure to read and has a reading list for further study. It will be welcomed by seekers and sufferers alike—that is by all of us.

Contents

Introduction

So much is being written about health matters these days and there are any number of opinions about what is good or bad for us. Whilst there is a great deal of disagreement there seems to be a consensus that lifestyle and diet affect our ability to enjoy good health. As a homoeopath and natural medicine practitioner I find that there is one area which has been greatly neglected in regard to health and well-being. It is that optimistic philosophy and understanding which takes account the meaning of life and what happens when our life on Earth finishes. This book is an endeavour to give some hope and encouragement to those who have a fear of death and who have avoided any consideration of this and the wider implications of their dis-ease or lack of harmony.

In my role as a homoeopathic practitioner I often pose the question 'Do you have any idea what happens when you die?' Sometimes such a query is unnecessary, at others it is inappropriate, but from a holistic health viewpoint it is most important. Once an individual knows what he or she is doing on Earth, and why, then that person can more easily come to terms with their problem and deal with it more effectively.

The answers to the question vary enormously. Some people, thanks to parental or other influences, are brought up to believe a particular religion and they are very clear about what is going to happen to them. The Christian seeks salvation. The Buddhist is taught to seek Nirvana. The Hindu aspires to union with the Beloved. Each is the same. I take the view that any faith that gives comfort or purpose is good but I am sometimes dismayed by the sort of response which runs along the lines 'I have not really thought about it' or, worse still, 'There is nothing'. On other occasions the reply indicates a definite fear of either thinking or talking about it and I hope that this volume will do something to help those people who are, perhaps, wondering about the whence, whither and why of our existence.

Many of our sense organs are very limited. The human ear responds only to the sounds within a frequency range of 30 to 16,000 cycles. Animals and birds do rather better than that. There are about 50 octaves of electromagnetic radiation yet our eyes pick up less than 1 octave. Our ideas and concepts of life are usually restricted to the 5 physical senses and I refer to these physical limitations because we live in a world of illusion. There is a much larger world out there than one can imagine—a super-sensible world. Super-sensible means above the physical. Some of us will know this as telepathy, clairvoyance, some other form of extra sensory perception or, simply, as intuition.

We are not just a physical body. If you look closely at any living object you may see the field of energy which surrounds it. It is the etheric body. The light has to be right and your eyes have to be relaxed in a particular way in order to see this. It is like a blueprint of the physical body. There are other bodies, beyond the etheric body and surrounding it, but I will leave that subject for the time being. I mention it now to make the point that we are not simply a bunch of molecules, strung together in some haphazard way, to be manipulated by scientists and doctors.

Scientists might know all about the structure of a golf ball but it would tell them nothing about the rules of golf or of its attraction for so many people. How does one measure, scientifically, the beauty of a sunset for example? There is a limit to the scientific approach; reason is an excellent guide but it is a poor master.

When I am encouraged to explain to a patient what I believe I try to do so in a few minutes. If they show some interest I might then refer that person to an appropriate book. Recently a patient, who benefited greatly from this sort of discussion, suggested I should write down my thoughts on the subject and hence this book.

The reader might well wonder who am I to tell them what happens when a person dies and it is a question which is difficult to answer convincingly. I can only say that, apart from what I have read and experienced in this life, the knowledge also comes from inside. For the sceptic there is nothing I can say which will prove that the essence of what follows, on the topic of life after death, is correct. However, anybody who takes the trouble to investigate, with an open mind, what is collectively known as The Ancient Wisdom cannot help but be persuaded about immortality. By Ancient Wisdom I mean the information contained in collections of books and documents held by many spiritually based societies or even in the spiritual section of most ordinary libraries. These are available to anybody with an enquiring mind.

Essentially we have to understand that we are, indeed, immortal and that so called death is really a change of form which enables us to leave the physical vehicle for a period of rest and recuperation. The collected evidence indicates pretty strongly that we may expect to return to Earth, after a suitable rest, in another body.

Undesirable as that my seem we have, apparently, all done it countless times but most of us have no recollection of our earlier lives once we are here again in another physical body. This is often in circumstances which many of us would certainly not have chosen at a conscious level! More on that a little later but, meanwhile, this is what the poet John Masefield said about it when he wrote his creed, parts of which I quote below:

A Creed

I hold that when a person dies
His soul returns again to earth;
Arrayed in some new flesh-disguise,
Another mother gives him birth.
With sturdier limbs and brighter brain
The old soul takes the roads again.

Such is my belief and trust;
This hand, this hand that holds the pen
Has many a hundred times been dust
And turned as dust to dust again;
These eyes of mine have blinked and shone
In Thebes, in Troy, in Babylon.

All that I rightly think or do,
Or make or spoil, or bless or blast,

Is curse or blessing justly due
For sloth or effort in the past.
My life's a statement of the sum
Of vice indulged, or overcome.

And as I wander on the roads
I shall be helped and healed and blessed;
Kind words shall cheer and be as goads
To urge to heights before unguessed.
My road shall be the road I made,
All that I gave shall be repaid.

So shall I fight, so shall I tread,
In this long war beneath the stars;
So shall a glory wreathe my head,
So shall I faint and show the scars,
Until this case, this clogging mould,
Be smithied all to kingly gold.

Before going on with my thoughts on our reasons for being here and of the life which follows I would like to say a little bit about orthodox medicine, suppression of disease, the role of food in good health, homoeopathy, breathing, holistic treatment and some of the differences between the gentle approach and that of orthodoxy.

CHAPTER 1.

Orthodoxy versus Holistic Medicine

There is a great difference in the approach to healing in the two systems. The holistic (whole-istic) approach is gentler and treats the patient at every level—spiritually, mentally, emotionally and physically. Orthodoxy, in general terms, is concerned with treating symptoms and has been likened to a plumber finding a leak and plugging it rather than reviewing the whole system.

It is an unfortunate fact of life that most orthodox general practitioners have a heavy workload and, as a consequence, they are not always able to devote time to listening to the patient's problems. The holistic practitioner is quite often able to help a patient simply by allowing sufficient time to do this.

To understand the gentler or holistic approach one must first know a little bit more about orthodox (allopathic) medicine. Whilst two centuries ago it was a blend of crude science, myth and superstition, today it is overwhelmingly scientific. It is so scientific and specialised that the individual with serious health problems is quite likely to be put in the hands of a specialist. The expertise of the specialist is usually concentrated in dealing with just one aspect of illness and sometimes this makes it difficult for the whole picture to be seen—an inability to see the wood for the trees. By contrast the holistic approach, which involves getting an overall picture of the ‘wood’, can frequently identify the real cause of the dis-ease.

There is a point of view which says that modern medicine, as we know it, has done little to cure or prevent disease when compared with the advantages conferred on society by good sanitation, improved housing, smaller families and other social improvements. It is true to say that a handful of drug innovations, such as antibiotics, have made a difference to life expectancy. However, I think it is wrong to believe that these innovations are responsible for saving the many millions of lives one might imagine. It is well known that killer infectious diseases were fast disappearing before drugs were available to cure them. Even tuberculosis was eradicated much more by social conditions than by drugs. The problem now is disease brought about by the over-use of drugs and antibiotics.

In general terms orthodox medicine tends to see every new case, especially of chronic disease, as a chance event. If a person develops cancer or gallstones or has some obscure disease then it is usually considered bad luck. The connection with what has gone before is often ignored. In an individual you might see a disease that manifested 10 years ago which we can call disease A. 5 years later the same individual appears in front of his doctor with another disease—let’s call it disease B. When he appears in front of his doctor today with disease C it is unlikely that the doctor will be aware of the thread connecting those 3 conditions. Probably it was the suppression of disease A which led to the foundation of disease B and the suppression of disease B which later resulted in disease C.

An example of this connection between various diseases might be that of a child fed with cow's milk. This can result in poor gut flora and possibly a zinc deficiency. Because of the poor gut flora and inability to deal with dairy products catarrh might result. In later years poor gut flora might result in constipation and a build-up of toxins. Tonsillitis could develop and this would likely be treated with antibiotics. If this proves unhelpful the tonsils are likely to be removed. This action, whilst resolving the immediate problem, might in the long term make the overall situation worse. Later in life appendicitis could develop and the appendix then removed. In the following years one might expect irritable bowel syndrome with its attendant problems and eventually arthritis might appear or, worse still, cancer.

CHAPTER 2.

Orthodoxy and Suppressive Treatment

Drugs and surgery are both suppressive treatments. Suppression equals a reduction of the vital force (or life force as it is sometimes called). This results in disease becoming chronic because the body is unable to throw off the toxic overload. The famous naturopath, Dr. Lindlahr stated that… 'Every acute disease is the result of a cleansing and healing effort on the part of nature'. When nature tries to show her hand by giving us a cold or a fever most people reach for an aspirin and immediately suppress this healing attempt. This is the orthodox way of doing things.

I recently came across a story which illustrates disease suppression in a dramatic way. It goes like this and is entitled:

'We Did Our Best'.

'A young man developed a sore throat. He went to his physician who prescribed penicillin for the inflammation. The sore throat promptly disappeared. Three days later he developed itching and hives all over his body. A physician correctly diagnosed a penicillin reaction and prescribed anti-histamines. The hives went away!

However, the anti-histamines caused the patient to be drowsy and he cut his hand whilst at work. He went to the company nurse who put some anti-bacterial salve on the injury. Unhappily, the salve contained penicillin which caused the hives to return.

Recognising a possible serious reaction to penicillin for the second time his doctor then prescribed cortisone. The hives disappeared once more.

The patient then developed abdominal pains and noticed blood on his stools. The correct diagnosis was made of a bleeding peptic ulcer brought on by the cortisone. Sadly, as the patient failed to respond to standard measures to correct the haemorrhage, the next course of action indicated was a partial gastrectomy. The surgery was successful. The stomach pains diminished and the bleeding stopped.

However, as the patient had previously lost so much blood due to haemorrhaging and during the surgery, a blood transfusion was indicated. He was given 2 pints of blood. Unhappily, he contracted hepatitis from the transfusion.

Being young and vital he recovered from the hepatitis but at the point of insertion of the transfusion needle a painful red swelling appeared indicating a probable infection. Having had previous bad experience with penicillin the drug of choice was now tetracycline. This was given and the infection promptly subsided.

Disruption of the intestinal flora by the tetracycline caused painful abdominal spasms and severe diarrhoea so the patient was given an antispasmodic type drug. The diarrhoea and spasms subsided.

Unfortunately the drug was in the belladonna or muscle relaxant group of drugs which relaxed the smooth muscles all over his body. The effect of the muscle relaxant on his eyes impaired the patient 's vision.... He drove his car into a tree and was killed instantly.'

This is reputed to be a true story and, if it isn't it certainly could be! It shows that the use of modern drugs and surgery is not always the answer despite the very best intentions.

The medical establishment has little time for unorthodoxy although it has to be said that times are changing and it is encouraging to note that a number of conventional doctors are now showing a lot in interest in holistic therapies.

Some of my natural medicine colleagues are very opposed to orthodoxy but my personal belief is that orthodox medicine cannot be dismissed so easily. The gentle approach does not have all the answers. I know that if I get run over I shall be only too pleased to receive orthodox treatment including surgery.

In the area of surgery and microsurgery there have been brilliant achievements. I am not personally in favour of transferring a heart from one body to another but it is a difficult line to draw. Some of the orthodox technical know-how is very valuable and we must take account of some of the diagnostic procedures available to it. I think the two approaches must be blended, where appropriate, for the benefit of those who are unwell.

CHAPTER 3.

Homoeopathy

Homoeopathy is just one of the many holistic approaches to disease. To many people it presents a baffling and unscientific collection of contradictions because it uses poisons to cure, toxins to detoxify, and dilutes drugs so much that the original substance is untraceable in any scientific analysis.

The origins of homoeopathy go back to 1810 when a German physician, Dr. Samuel Hahnemann, first proposed a new system of medicine as an alternative to the orthodox practices of the day. These included bloodletting and purging, which Hahnemann thought were too harsh, and often weakened patients more than did their illnesses. By contrast, the new system was to be based on gentler ways of helping the body to cure itself.

Hahnemann's ideas were inspired by the discovery that a herbal remedy for malaria—cinchona tree bark—produced symptoms of the disease, such as headache and fever, when taken by a healthy person. He concluded that symptoms were the body's way of fighting illness and that medicines which produced the same symptoms as an illness could aid recovery. (It was later discovered that cinchona bark contains quinine, the first drug used against malaria).

Hahnemann's ideas were, in effect, a re-discovery of an ancient principle first expressed by the Greek physician Hippocrates in the fifth century BC. It can be summed up by the Latin 'similia similibus curentur' meaning 'let likes cure like'. Hahnemann called the new system Homoeopathy meaning 'like disease' in contrast to conventional medicine, which he termed Allopathy meaning 'against disease' since it uses medicines to suppress or prevent symptoms.

The law of dual effect—that of action and reaction—applies throughout nature and is the very foundation of healing science. It relates to and governs every phenomenon of health, disease and cure. What is commonly called a crisis, acute reaction or acute disease is, in reality, nature's attempt to establish health. Every agent affecting the human organism produces two effects: a first, temporary effect, and a second, lasting effect. The second, lasting effect, is always contrary to the first, temporary effect.

For example, the first temporary effect of cold water applied to the skin results in blood going to the interior of the body. However, in order to compensate for the local depletion nature responds by sending greater quantities back to the surface resulting in increased warmth and better surface circulation. Conversely, the first effect of a hot bath is to draw blood to the surface but the second effect sends the blood back to the interior, leaving the surface bloodless and chilled. Stimulants produce their deceptive effects by consuming the reserve stores of vital energy in the organism. This in inevitably followed by weakness and exhaustion in exact proportion to the previous excitation. The first effect of relaxation and sleep is weakness and half consciousness; the second effect, however, is an increase in vitality.

This dual effect applies to all drug action. The first

temporary, violent effect of poisonous drugs is usually due to nature's efforts to overcome and eliminate these substances. For instance if one takes a purgative the body will respond by trying to throw it out of the system and thus the first effect is to cause a bowel movement. The second, lasting effect, is less welcome as continued use of purgatives is likely to cause constipation. This second effect is due to the retention of drug poisons in the system and their destructive action on the organism.

In theory and in practice allopathy considers the first effect only and ignores the lasting after-effects of drugs and surgical operations. It administers remedies whose first effect is contrary to the disease condition. Therefore, in accordance with the law of action and reaction, which are equal but opposite (well nearly equal according to the latest findings in quantum physics!), the second and lasting effect of such remedies must be similar to the disease condition.

Everyday experiences indicate the validity of this thinking. The long term use of laxatives has already been mentioned—where the temporary irritation and overstimulation of the sensitive membranes of the digestive organs are followed by corresponding weakness and exhaustion. If this procedure is repeated often enough it becomes habitual. Another example is the continued use of stimulants and tonics. Eventually this can cause complete exhaustion and a reduction of physical and mental ability.

Opiates, sedatives and hypnotics may give temporary relief but, if due to constitutional causes, the result will be a worsening of the original condition and possible addiction to the drug. Each drug breeds new disease symptoms which are in turn cured by other poisons and the vicious circle is continued.

On the other hand, the teaching and practice of homoeopathy is fully in harmony with the law of dual effect (action and reaction). Letting 'likes cure like' it administers remedies in minute doses whose first, but temporary effect, is similar to the disease condition and whose second but lasting effect must be contrary to the disease condition and thus curative.

Hahnemann thought that small doses of homoeopathic remedies would be safer than large ones whilst still being effective. He spent many years experimenting on himself and his family and friends with a wide range of natural substances in dilute forms. His approach was 'holistic' for it concentrated on the whole person—spiritual, mental, emotional and, physical. The homoeopathic remedies were aimed at restoring the body's natural balance and boosting the vital force thus enabling it to fight disease.

Over the years, Hahnemann, by close observation and experiment, established the following 3 principles of homoeopathy:

1) A medicine, which in large doses produces symptoms of a disease, will in small doses cure that disease.

2) By extreme dilution the medicine's curative properties are improved and all the poisonous or undesirable side effects are lost.

3) Homoeopathic medicines are prescribed individually by the study of the whole person which includes temperament, emotions and general constitution.

To give the reader an idea of how this works let me give a brief summary of the provings for 3 well known remedies:

Coffee in excess will produce excitability, sleeplessness, headaches, restlessness, palpitations and a variety of other symptoms. In homoeopathic form, for certain individuals, it can be used to calm and aid sleep.

Arsenic in significant doses would cause restlessness, burning pains, fear, cold sweat, thirst, diarrhoea, etc. A person demonstrating some of these symptoms who fits this homoeopathic 'picture' could be cured by arsenic in homoeopathic potency.

Deadly nightshade or belladonna in significant doses will cause heat, redness, throbbing or burning pains and dilated pupils, amongst other symptoms, but unlike arsenic no thirst, no anxiety or fear. In homoeopathic strength it can be used to restore somebody demonstrating these symptoms.

In short ALLOPATHY treats symptoms, looks on microbes as a cause, names diseases, gives large doses, is suppressive, and tests on animals.

HOMOEOPATHY treats the whole person, acknowledges the presence of microbes, does not name diseases, gives small doses, stimulates self healing, and tests on humans.

The average patient who visits a homoeopath for the first time is often somewhat mystified by the ensuing interview because most homoeopaths take a rather different approach to the patient than does the average orthodox doctor. A good homoeopath will have a very personal approach to the patient because he is concerned with the whole person rather than with the clinical symptoms of a specific disease. He is concerned with treating the patient and not the disease.

Homoeopathic philosophy accepts that there is a basic force within the patient often referred to as the life force. The absence of it would be seen as the difference between a living and a dead body. The life force is the very essence of the patient and it is this force that controls the health of the individual. Disease is dis-ease; a condition in which the body is out of harmony with itself and this elusive force is diminished.

The reasons for this dis-harmony may be due, simply, to the strains and stresses of modern life taking their toll. It might be due to an accidental injury or progressive poisoning of the body with toxins of one sort or another. Perhaps it is the outcome of long term drug treatment or it might be due to an inherited weakness or miasm as it is called in homoeopathic terms. It might be a combination of many things.

The homoeopath acknowledges that the human body is basically a self healing mechanism and the less interference this mechanism suffers the better it will function. The life force has enormous potential and the homoeopathic remedy needs to resonate with it in order to stimulate the body to heal itself. As previously stated, essential to the administration of homoeopathic remedies is the principle of dilution or, rather, potentisation. Very minute doses of the original substance are used and in some mysterious way the more diluted the remedy the more potent it becomes. Is is this subtle energy which influences or resonates with the vital force and encourages the body to heal itself.

To the patient homoeopathy is a commitment to a real cure. The patient has to realise that he cannot push all the responsibility for a cure on to the practitioner but must work with him to climb the slope to recovery. Modern homoeopathy is perhaps very close to spiritual medicine. It is a blend of science and magic.

There is still a lot which is not fully understood about the workings of homoeopathy but most homoeopaths see enough evidence of remarkable changes in their patients to know that they are using a system which, by and large, gives excellent results. For all that the more one knows the more one realises how much more there is to know. In some ways it is a bit like electricity in the sense that we know how to use it quite successfully but nobody seems to know exactly what it is!

CHAPTER 4.

Living to Eat or Eating to Live?

The area of nutrition is one which has been more or less ignored in orthodox medicine until recently. At the time of writing it does seem that the government is at last turning its attention to the importance of diet and preventive medicine so we should not be too discouraged. I cannot resist the opportunity of expressing my view that a wholefood diet, rich in vegetables and with a minimum of animal foods and especially animal fats, is much better than one full of refined sugar products, processed foods and the flesh of animals.

The food we eat is very important. We are what we eat or rather what we absorb. There is an interesting book about diet and delinquency by Alexander Schauss. The thrust of it is that many criminals are not born bad but simply commit crimes because they feel bad. The reason they feel so bad is because they eat so badly. To cut a long story short they eat quantities of junk food, overloaded with sugar and additives of one sort or another with the result that they are frequently nutritionally deficient or simply suffering with hypoglycaemia (low blood sugar). Such mineral deficiencies and abnormal sugar levels can influence mood and cause all kinds of aberrant behaviour.

Organically grown foods have a greater vitality (life force) than fruits and vegetables conventionally produced using fertilizers, pesticides, etc. Results of some recent scientific tests which measure the units of light emitted from food show that organically produced food gives consistently higher readings than those grown conventionally. This light energy is thought to be stored in the DNA during photosynthesis when plants are busy converting sunlight and water to organic material. The light is transmitted continuously by every cell. The theory is that the higher the level of light energy a cell emits the greater its vitality and the more potential for the transfer of that energy to someone eating the food. In short, for increased life force or vitality, it helps to eat organically grown foods.

In my experience there are some commonly used foods which many of my patients have eliminated from their diets with remarkable benefits. These are milk, milk based products, wheat and wheat based products. Refined sugar and salt are also to be discouraged.

According to some nutritionists one of the prime problems with milk is that it makes for poor intestinal absorption because it neutralises stomach acid, leaving protein only partly digested. Milk forms an excessive and unhealthy mucus in the digestive tract which, combined with other food residues, hardens to inhibit the absorption of minerals and other nutrients. Milk encourages alkali forming putrefactive bacteria to live in the intestines, again creating conditions unsuitable for mineral absorption. The high calcium content of milk itself is frequently not absorbed for this reason.

It is worth bearing in mind that cows discourage their calves from consuming milk after weaning. In short, cow's milk is good for young calves as human milk is good for young babies. Once beyond babyhood milk is not a useful food—especially cow's milk for humans! In cow's milk, casein, the main protein, is poorly digested by humans and additionally may contain hormones secreted by the cow's pituitary gland, including growth hormone which is not destroyed by processing. Such milk can lead to unnatural growth in children.

The mucus forming tendency of milk in connection with the intestines applies equally to the mucous membranes of the nose, sinuses, etc, causing catarrh, hay fever, fallopian tube blockages, eustachian tube blockages and so on. Remember that cheese is concentrated milk and has a high salt content.

Milk encourages sodium (salt) to enter the cells and the eventual result of this is energy depletion. A sodium excess in the diet over a long period overwhelms the mechanism in the body to deal with this excess and results in a rise in acidity and sodium concentration. The two tend to go hand in hand. The mineral magnesium gets excluded from the cells and as a consequence the sodium 'pump' mechanism can no longer work efficiently. The resulting intracellular magnesium deficiency depresses the sodium 'pump' still further and a vicious circle is created. Potassium is also lost from the cells under these conditions and trace elements such as zinc, manganese and chromium tend to be denied access to the cells.

A lot of different minerals are critical to the mechanism which controls blood sugar levels. Calcium metabolism is also severely affected and blood sugar levels are very closely related to the blood calcium level. If there is a drop in blood sugar level, because of the drop in blood calcium level, the individual will suffer a loss of energy. The normal response would be for the pancreas and adrenal glands to go into action but if there is a lack of trace minerals in the body they will have difficulty in doing so and pancreatic and adrenal exhaustion may eventually result.

Sugary foods such as cakes, chocolate bars, sweets, biscuits, pastries, etc. and stimulant beverages such as tea, coffee, 'coke', etc. cause the blood sugar to rise initially (hence the craving for them) but the level falls quickly and causes severe mineral loss. Another vicious circle begins and progressively stronger stimulants are needed to pick-up the individual lacking energy. Sometimes, when the blood sugar level drops very low, odd patterns of behaviour can occur such as bursts of temper, tearfulness and so on. Conditions including the pre-menstrual syndrome, migraine, asthma, epilepsy, colitis, irritable bowel syndrome may be provoked or become more severe at these times.

Intestinal stasis is one of the results of eating gluten containing foods, especially wheat products such as bread, pasta, pastries, and is due to the glue-like quality it assumes when poorly digested and mixed with mucus and other liquids in the digestive tract. The gluey substance adheres to and lines the walls of the colon making for poor absorption. Peristaltic movement is less effective and the stasis is self perpetuating. Putrifying bacteria, invading the static mass, contributes towards auto-intoxication. Diverticuli may develop in the bowel thus providing a home for more bacteria with direct access into the bloodstream for these toxins.

I realise that avoiding wheat and dairy products is

not very easy but the rewards are considerable; if one cannot avoid them totally then it so worth minimising the intake of these items as well as refined sugar and salt.

CHAPTER 5.

Vegetarian—to Be or Not to Be?

There are many discussions about what is 'natural' for human beings to eat. If one looks at the diet of mammals there are two groups. Flesh-eating animals such as dogs, cats, tigers and lions; and vegetarian animals like cows, bulls, horses, camels, giraffes and even the mighty elephants.

When comparing their physical features the flesh-eating animals have long teeth to tear the raw animal flesh from the bones whilst the vegetarian animals have flat teeth for grinding vegetable food. Meat-eating animals have rough tongues to lick flesh from the bone and sharp strong claws to catch and kill their prey unlike the vegetarian creatures. Interestingly, too, they have excellent night vision for hunting whilst the vegetarians have more difficulty in seeing after dusk.

Less obvious are differences in the intestines. In the meat-eating group these are generally only 2 to 3 times the body length thus facilitating the rapid passage of the meat eaten before it has time to putrefy. In vegetarian animals, the intestines are generally 6 to 7 times the length of their bodies because the contents need to be retained for a longer period. Vegetarian creatures have digestive enzymes in their saliva and begin digesting food whilst it is still in the mouth. They also have a different pH, in both their stomachs and saliva, than the flesh eating creatures. (The pH is a measure of acidity or alkalinity where pH7 is neutral. Below pH7 acidity increases and above it alkalinity increases). Starch digestion is thought to require alkaline conditions whereas protein (meat) digestion requires acid conditions.

Humans have flat teeth for grinding like the vegetarian animals and smoother tongues than the carnivores who tend to gulp their food without much chewing. Humans are (usually!) without sharp claws and their vision is not very good after dusk. Generally speaking human intestines are about 26 feet long or 6 to 7 times as long as the trunks of their bodies. The pH of human saliva is similar to vegetarian animals and, like them, the saliva contains digestive enzymes. In these respects of physical design humans certainly have a lot in common with the non meat-eating animals.

If one looks carefully at the differences in behaviour between meat-eating and vegetarian animals at a zoo it will be observed that the meat eaters can be fierce and aggressive. The cages of the meat eaters will smell strongly in line with everything else that exudes from their bodies. The vegetarian animals, on the other hand, are relatively calm and gentle.

When an animal is killed its body immediately starts to decay. Anybody eating meat is literally eating dead matter. This rapid decaying process is one reason why animal matter leaves so much toxic material in the systems of those consuming it. Vegetables may dehydrate after they are chopped but it will take quite some time for those vegetables to decay.

Some people argue that is possible to find killed

animals to eat that are healthy but, at the moment of slaughter, all kinds of undesirable toxins, and hormones such as adrenalin, permeate the body tissues. These residues remain in the meat which is later consumed. Because human intestines are so long the decayed flesh cannot be digested and pass though before putrefying. The body tries to filter out toxins through the eliminative system, including perspiration and breath, and it is this process which can cause foul perspiration odour. However, not all toxins will be eliminated. Those remaining will contribute to the overall toxic load in the body which is the precursor of dis-ease.

Carnivorous humans point out that meat is a rich source of protein. This is true; but it is known that humans do not need such a concentrated protein to metabolise the body. Vegetarians believe that protein should be as close to its natural source as possible. It is plentiful, in simpler form and easier to digest in soya beans, in lentils, in avocados, in nuts and in seeds such as pumpkin and sunflower. In any event the need for large amounts of protein is much exaggerated in the West and the problem is often an excess of it rather than insufficiency.

Vegetarians claim to have bodies that are healthier, more supple and less tense than those of their animal eating counterparts. Various studies have been conducted on the benefits of vegetarianism. These have shown very positive effects but for some people more 'scientific' evidence is required. Perhaps, in the future, trials on a grand scale will provide the sort of evidence that is needed?

It could be argued that it would be difficult to convince an Eskimo, whose diet is primarily meat, that he should be vegetarian. The Eskimo would starve without it. Obviously a vegetarian diet in such an environment, where even grass does not grow, would be impossible. It is interesting to note, however, that the average life span of an Eskimo is less than 30 years. The Hunzas of Pakistan whose diet is primarily vegetarian live to a very old age with recorded ages of 110 not uncommon. People who eat a lot of meat are often concerned that they will be unable to keep up their strength without it but horses, oxen, bulls and elephants to not seem to have a problem!

The violence in our society poses a threat to its very existence. There are those who believe that the meat diet is part of that violence. It involves killing, often in hideous circumstances, and on a grand scale. Anybody who has witnessed how animals die in a slaughterhouse cannot help but be influenced by it. There is a curious double standard in that many people who would be unable to carry out or even witness such events are happy to allow other people to do it on their behalf. Equally many pet lovers will go to great lengths to prevent cruelty to some animals but at the same time encourage a trade which brings about the deaths of countless lambs, calves and cows. One wonders what the difference is between a cow's life and that of a cat? There are many who believe that there will always be wars so long as man continues to treat animals inhumanely.

When we eat vegetables we are also destroying something; but we have to eat, and the plant is not as developed as the animal in the expression of its consciousness. The more developed the expression of that consciousness, in a particular form of life, the more pain is felt when it is destroyed. Cutting off the branch of a tree causes less pain than cutting off the limb of an animal. Studies have shown that plants do experience pain but it is not considered to be on the same level as that experienced by warm-blooded creatures with a developed nervous system.

The Hindu scriptures talk about '...consciousness sleeping in the mineral kingdom, dreaming in plant life and awakening in animal life'. It is a similar consciousness in all but functioning at different levels. For instance in animals we see instinct functioning and in humans there is intelligence.

There are other considerations and these are the economic and ecological ones. There is certainly an unequal distribution of food in the world and the starvation experienced in some parts is sometimes blamed on overpopulation there. There is a point of view, however, which is that the resources we have are adequate if we are all willing to share them equally. According to some sources it needs 16 pounds of grain to be fed to a bull in order to get one pound of meat. This amount of grain would go a lot further if fed directly to humans. Looked at another way, an acre of land used for grain production gives 5 times as much protein as an acre used for producing meat. An acre of beans or lentils gives 10 times as much protein, and an acre of vegetables 15 times as much protein.

Meat is a rich source of minerals and the smell of meat cooking is a very appetising one for many people. It has to be borne in mind that the meat industry would be doomed without the present custom so these are considerations to be borne in mind when weighing the arguments! It is for individuals to decide where their priorities lie. For those who do wish to consider becoming vegetarian I believe the transition should be made gradually. Initially one could start by avoiding red meat whilst continuing to eat fowl and fish for some time. Later, fowl can be left out of the diet, leaving fish and eggs—eventually graduating to vegetarian food only. A body which is used to eating flesh may still demand it in the same way that the body of a smoker, who has relinquished the habit, craves nicotine. The cells remember it so there may be some difficulty at first. However, as your body becomes less toxic it will become easier, and you may find yourself crossing the road to avoid a butcher's shop as the odour emanating from it may be something which you can no longer tolerate.

Whatever we decide to eat it is as well to do so with a feeling of gratitude and to bear in mind the words of Mahatma Gandhi who said 'The earth has enough for everyone's need, but not enough for everyone's greed.'

CHAPTER 6.

A Word on Breathing

Since breathing is central to all the functions of the body it is important that we understand how to breathe deeply. Proper breathing is much neglected and overlooked and yet it has a profound effect on health. It can enhance vitality and well-being and also bring tranquillity and harmony into our lives. Breathing influences us physically, emotionally and mentally.

Since many people spend their entire lives using only a small part of their lungs it is worth spending a few minutes to practise the correct technique. If you use only a small part of your lungs there will always be a residue of stale air left that can eventually become toxic with consequent ill effects throughout the system.

Here is a technique you may like to try:

Start by sitting comfortably on a firm chair in a relaxed fashion but keep the spine straight. Some people may prefer to lie flat on the floor instead of sitting. In the latter case a folded blanket or rug beneath the body is helpful to ensure comfort and relaxation. An extra folded blanket under the top half of the body from waist to head facilitates expansion of the chest and helps the free flow of air.

Close your eyes and inwardly observe the breath flowing in and out for a few minutes. Connect to this rhythm and sense the breath becoming softer, deeper and slower. After a while become aware of the phases of the breath:

How the inhalation starts at the base of the lungs with the gentle movement of the diaphragm.

How it then moves to the middle of the lungs as the rib cage rises upwards and outwards.

And, finally, how the breath rises to the very top of the lungs with a quiet, smooth movement. The upper ribs slide under the collar bones and sideways towards the armpits.

The exhalation follows the same pattern, starting at the base and working upwards as the breath quietly leaves the body.

Breathing in this deep, conscious manner should never be forced but done with quiet concentration. As you continue the breath will naturally deepen and the lung capacity will expand.

After a few minutes of being aware of these movements visualise the breath as light. On the inward breath take the light to the heart centre (the area around the centre of your chest). On the outward breath see the light as rays of the sun radiating to every part of your body and filling every cell with light. If you practise this you will become aware of the form and shape of your body as light.

Ten minutes a day of quiet concentration on the art

of breathing will bring enormous benefits. It may encourage a deeper study of the connection between the breath and the more subtle levels of our being.

At another level the conscious breathing-in of the light, and conscious breathing-out of love to mankind, is immensely valuable. This deep rhythmic breathing does more than affect the body. Seen clairvoyantly, the person breathing-in, and being aware of this divine breath, is strengthening his soul and causing it to radiate a great light. Such a light is able to traverse the world and, indeed, the universe.

CHAPTER 7.

Healing

We are all healers. However, some people seem unaware of this whereas others make an effort to develop their healing ability. When a child falls down and hurts some part of its anatomy the first thing the mother does is to pick up the child and probably rub a soothing hand over the injured part. This is healing. She does it automatically. How often have you put a hand out to touch a friend in need of comfort? This, too, is healing.

It is our duty to keep our physical bodies healthy by living in harmony with both natural and divine law. When these laws are broken through some weakness in ourselves, we suffer. The body is of the Creator and it needs to be treated with respect and consideration; to be loved. If we are to do this we must not overwork, overstrain, overfeed or over-indulge ourselves in any way. It really is our duty to care for the physical vehicle by treating it gently and wisely.

Every physical disability arises from some disharmony in the soul, some lack of balance or some emotional conflict. The idea is, perhaps, unpalatable to many of us. We do not like to admit that our sickness is due to some disharmony or fault in ourselves. Lack of harmony in our thoughts and in our lives brings dis-ease; harmony brings health. We must let go of all resentment, fear or criticism.

The natural physical instinct is to fear but we need

to learn that no harm can touch the real person within. There is nothing to fear except fear itself. If we have full confidence in the Creator light will flow through our being and all darkness will be eliminated. Remember—where there is light there can be no darkness.

Basically all healing is the intake into the body of the eternal sun, the light. We need to call upon this light, breathe it in, see it and live consciously in it. This light has the power to control the cells of the physical body. We are so encumbered with our heavy physical bodies, and material life is so strong, that we can be forgiven for overlooking the fact that the very cells and tissues of our bodies can be re-created.

Trained healers work in a variety of ways. There are many techniques but the important ingredient is unconditional love. It is helpful to visualise the healing energy coming through from a higher source. Simply using one's own energy can be depleting which is both undesirable and unnecessary.

In contact healing, that is when the person requiring help is with you, one simple technique is to imagine (visualise in your mind) light or energy coming from the sun. Imagine this force pouring into your body and then think of yourself as a transformer converting it into a form which is acceptable to the person who has asked for help. Visualise the light permeating your entire being and then going out via your hands so that the flow can be directed to the required area.

This same healing thought (thought is energy) can be used at a distance. You do not have to have a person next to you to give them healing. Simply visualise the person to whom you wish to send a healing thought and that healing energy will be with the person immediately. Distance is of no importance. It is like saying a prayer for somebody you love and it is instantaneous!

As indicated above, the technique is not so vital as the unconditional love and the simple, but clear, thought which goes into it. It is worth having a mind picture or visualisation which you can readily use at any convenient moment when the need is there.

The concept of reincarnation (more on this later) has already been advanced and so far as healing is concerned we ought not to separate one life from another. Instead we should try to look upon the chain of incarnations as one continuous story or think of them as chapters in a long book. The disharmony might be so subtle that is would take a seer to perceive it. We frequently break spiritual laws by overstraining our physical, emotional or mental bodies. This common cause, often disregarded, results in a lack of balance and harmony. Most of us are guilty of it on a fairly regular basis! Is it any wonder we become ill from time to time?

Where does one stand with healing if bodily suffering and sickness are due to the outworking of karma? Karma is an eastern word used to describe the inexorable law of cause and effect. In biblical terms it is covered by the phrase 'as one sows so one reaps'. Is it right to try to help sufferers to overcome such karma by giving spiritual healing? I think it is. We have to do our best to help and heal those who ask for or need our assistance.

The parable of the good Samaritan illustrates the point. In that parable Jesus advises us to love our neighbours as ourselves. When asked by a lawyer

'...who is my neighbour?', Jesus talked about a man who had been stripped, beaten and left half dead by robbers on the road from Jerusalem to Jericho. This unfortunate was ignored by a priest and a Levite but greatly helped by the Samaritan who rendered every assistance.

What part has the patient to play in such healing? The patient is being offered a magnificent opportunity, which originates from his 'good karma', to rise above the affliction of body and soul. If the man is wise he will respond to the opportunity and endeavour to learn the lesson which is proffered. In this way, by aspiring to the highest instinct, the karma is thus worked out or transmuted.

What about the saints in the world, who undergo apparently dreadful suffering? One might wonder where the disharmony or conflict is in those souls? To find the cause of the suffering of today we would probably need to go back further than one life to find the answer. It might be the final outworking and 'balancing of the books' for some error in the long past.

All human life is governed by divine law and, necessary though it may be to endure pain whilst in a physical body, it is to be hoped we will do so with courage. The problems with which we are faced, if looked upon as an opportunity from which to learn wisdom, will be more easily borne. We have to remember that, in accordance with the law of cause and effect (karma), the sufferer has at some time sown the seed for the current experiences. Thus there is little point blaming the Creator (or anybody else for that matter!).

CHAPTER 8.

Holistic Treatment

Here are three cases which I believe are good examples of what I mean by holistic treatment and healing.

The first case concerns a woman who is now aged 39 whom I will call Anne. She first came to me about 6 years ago suffering with a recurrent candida (thrush) problem and she also complained of frequent headaches. Anne had tried a number of alternative therapies but none of them seem to have any lasting benefit.

During the initial interview it emerged that her social life was not very satisfactory and she was not happy at her work as a nursery nurse/teacher. She had a relationship with a divorced and rather embittered man who had remarkably violent and curious political views. He also appeared to be rather lazy and selfish. It was clear that this man was taking advantage of Anne's good nature and kindness and offering very little in return.

The current relationship appeared to be one of a series in which she was being exploited by her partner. Anne was really aware of this at a subconscious level and talking about it helped to remove her head from the sand as she put it. By making her aware of this at a conscious level she realised that her ostrich-like view of the situation had to change.

On the homoeopathic front I felt that a residue of a childhood illness might be blocking her recovery in some measure. Additionally, she needed a constitutional remedy to help boost her own self-healing capacity.

Various homoeopathic remedies and supplements were prescribed over the following months but, more importantly I believe, our discussions during the first and subsequent consultations opened up a spiritual side which had been dormant for some time. Anne had drifted away from her particular church because she found it unsatisfactory for various reasons and was in a spiritual vacuum.

She acknowledged later that my suggestion of sending light or love to those people with whom she was in conflict, rather than hating them, had given her food for thought. She decided to end the unsatisfactory relationship and, additionally, as the spiritual side of her re-emerged her health problems improved.

Anne's dissatisfaction with her job was also a key issue and I encouraged here to pursue an interest in massage and aromatherapy. She did this with great enthusiasm and eventually gave up her work at the nursery school to become an excellent professional aromatherapist. Nowadays Anne is also involved in meditation, colour healing and a variety of new age interests. She is happy and to quote her.... 'is in harmony with life'.

Many people who seek complementary advice do so because they have had some bad experiences with orthodox medical treatment. This second case concerns a man of 55, whom I will call John, whose diabetes went undiagnosed until he was aged 51.

During an extensive initial interview it emerged that John had been a hypersensitive child whose parents had argued a good deal. The domestic scenes between his parents were very traumatic and left their mark on him. Around 21 he left the parental home to marry and set up on his own. In the following years he was very aware of how much the atmosphere of peace and tranquility at the home of his in-laws contrasted with the home he had left.

All went well with his life until about age 25 when he began experiencing unpleasant symptoms in the form of heavy perspiration and a prickling sensation in the genital area. This was coupled with feelings of intense irritation. On consulting his GP, who seemed puzzled by the condition, John volunteered that his father was diabetic and that he, too, had experienced similar unusual symptoms. This information did not seem of interest to the doctor and he sent John to a skin specialist. Within seconds of his examination the specialist made his diagnosis and John was informed, via his GP, that the problem was 'psychosomatic'.

The 'psychosomatic' condition persisted for 8 or 9 years despite repeated efforts to get further help from his medical advisors. He became what is known as a 'thick file case' or, in every day terms, a troublemaker! In his early 30s he experienced cramps in various limbs and was then referred by his GP to the National Hospital for Nervous Diseases. There 'amyotonia' was diagnosed, a lack of muscle tone for which no treatment was offered.

At age 35 John experienced a terrible pain in the left buttock which caused him to pass out. The doctor was called and diagnosed a 'slipped disc'. The doctor was called again 6 hours later and was alarmed to find that the 'slipped disc' was a massive embolism the left leg (a blocked artery). Some hours later in hospital his wife was informed that the leg might have to be amputated and that there was some doubt that John would survive the operation. In the event, after a 5 hour operation during which John had to be resuscitated, some of the blockage was removed.

Two days of intensive care followed and John was aware of waking up after this to a room 'filled with golden light' where 'everything seemed fresh and clean'. Additionally he said 'I was filled with a great love for my fellow men and especially for my immediate loved ones.'

After convalescing he returned to work, which had previously been approached with great enthusiasm and vigour, only to find that he now experienced abnormal fatigue. The problems in the genital area persisted and indeed worsened. His physical state deteriorated steadily over the next decade or so. Symptoms such as inability to climb stairs, mental drowsiness, reduced eyesight and general weariness all contributed to a very unsatisfactory life. At about 48 John's nervous system deteriorated sharply and he became blind.

At about this time, since it appeared his medical advisors where unable to think of anything else, he was directed to an allergy clinic. The doctor there was unable to come up with any allergen in particular but suggested that the weakness and fatigue were due to 'leaky adrenal glands'. He wrote to John's latest GP to this effect but test results later proved negative. This GP nonetheless maintained interest and John gave the doctor a list of all the illnesses he had experienced since birth. Presented with this the GP said that a test for diabetes was the next thing to do.

Needless to say the test proved positive. The sad part was that John, because of his father's diabetes, had been suggesting it as a cause for years! Within a relatively short time his metabolism was balanced and after 2 major eye operations his sight was restored. The non-diagnosis of diabetes for so many years had its consequences in the form of skin problems, diabetic neuropathy, poor sleep, high blood pressure and continued physical malaise resulting in a joyless existence.

When John had finished telling me his story, and after he had answered various questions I put to him, I was able to start him on a course of homoeopathic treatment. I was also able to suggest a number of supplements coupled with dietary changes which I felt would improve his general condition and feeling of well-being.

We talked of many things and there were some factors in his life which had been bottled up for many years. We discussed his life and spiritual matters including his near death experience. That interview put in motion a great spiritual change which, it seemed, had been waiting to happen. His earlier experience, during the recovery from the emergency operation on the embolism, was a taste of what was to come.

By forgiving himself, and by letting go of the guilt he felt over a particular matter, his atonement or at-one-ment with the Creator made a profound difference in his life. In subsequent visits the change in John was extraordinary. Fortunately he had always received great help and support from his wife and he was appreciative of this fact. His medical problems improved in some measure but, more importantly, there was a total change in his view of life. A calmer, serene, totally accepting individual emerged with a different set of values. The spiritual evolution continues today.

The third case concerns an attractive girl of 25. Clare, as I will call her, had a skin problem in the form of acne. Such a skin problem is not uncommon in people who, at a subconscious level, are not at peace with themselves.

Clare was one of 3 children born into a reasonably happy, hard-working household. There was some lack of closeness with her parents in the early years. She did not especially like school and her main interest from a young age was horses.

Clare had a steady boy friend from the age of about 16 and this relationship endured for about 5 years. She worked for one of the major banks and was well thought of by her employers. At 23 she became engaged to another man and it was generally a good relationship. On, the face of it everything in the garden was rosy and she and her fiancé eventually decided to share a house. Unhappily, soon after this, problems began to emerge. Something was lacking in this alliance and Clare was reluctant to finally tie the knot and get married.

At my suggestion a number of dietary changes were instituted and I prescribed various homoeopathic remedies, but, whilst the skin condition ameliorated in some measure, there was still room for improvement.

As I got to know Clare better I was able to touch on the whence, whither and why referred to at the beginning of this book. I loaned her a number of books on this subject. Clare found some of the information almost frightening to begin with but gradually her eyes were opened and her interest increased.

In the fullness of time she began to understand more about her purpose on Earth. Clare arrived at the conclusion that her engagement should be terminated and that her life was going to take a different turn. Whilst appreciating the financial rewards of life as a bank employee she was aware that it was not fulfilling her as she would have liked. She turned her attention to alternative therapies and started on a course of training as an aromatherapist.

The gradual unfolding of her understanding of the spiritual aspect of life has had a profound effect. She is now happier, more assured and at peace with herself. The acne has disappeared. She still consults me from time to time (mainly, I think to discuss esoteric matters!) and it is always a great pleasure to see her. Holistic healing personified in my view.

I was in my late 30s when I began to learn something of the whence, whither and why of my own existence. I had travelled the world to some extent and had enjoyed a reasonably successful commercial career for a number of years. It had allowed me to live in the Orient for quite a time followed by a stint in West Africa before I went to live in the Mediterranean area.

Things began to go wrong in my early 30s and there was a slow decline but I was about 38 when the major crisis occurred. My personal life was a disaster area; I was dissatisfied with my work and, by then, I had lost a great deal of money. When the lowest point came I was living in a rented room belonging to a farmer in the Provence area of France. It was a rather bleak, sparsely furnished room with a sink and a cold tap in one corner. A substantial contrast to the life I had experienced in the Far East some years previously. I had decided to live in Provence for a while, to think things out, but I was having great difficulty in obtaining any sort of job. I was quite happy to be a labourer but after being rejected by numerous potential employers for all sorts of menial jobs I was very nearly at the end of my tether. It was the final straw which was about to break the camel's back. My life, it seemed to me, had been a total failure. I was miserable and I blamed myself for a lot of the unhappiness I had left in my wake. Here I was in a foreign land, lonely and miles for anybody whom I might think of as a friend.

I felt the solution was to terminate my life and gave serious thought as to how I might do this. Two considerations held me back. One was the thought that my parents would somehow be notified about the discovery of my body and I was reluctant to inflict this further misery on them. The other was the knowledge, recently gained, that life is an eternal business and that even if I opted out of this incarnation I would eventually be back again in another body to face similar problems.

Looking back it hardly seems possible that I contemplated this matter so seriously but when one is sufficiently depressed and disheartened one does not think rationally. I do remember taking the telephone number of the Samaritan Organisation and I promised myself that I would speak to one of their number before I did the deed. That night I was literally on my knees and begging for help from 'whoever was up there'. I prayed (if that is the right word) for some sort of a break. I was a completely broken man.

Fortunately, the following day I did get a break and, to cut a long story short, managed to get a job as a dishwasher soon afterwards. That was a most important new beginning for me. It started me on a road of discovery and I spent the next few months working physically hard but doing a job which allowed my mind to soar in all sorts of directions. With the help of the Theosophical Society in Marseille I had access to numerous books dealing with various facets of the Ancient Wisdom and I learned a great deal.

My research confirmed that it would not have been a good idea to terminate my life prematurely. Had I done so it would, as I had suspected, simply have meant reincarnating to face the same problems in another body. Gradually I learned about the interconnection of all life and of the existence of the etheric, astral and mental bodies which are linked to our physical self. I realised how fortunate I was to be in an incarnation which was giving me the opportunity to learn. My life now had a purpose. I realised it was not enough simply to earn a living. I had to try to do something useful. It had been a long hard struggle but now, at last, I could see light at the end of the tunnel.

CHAPTER 9.

Reincarnation

The modern world appears confused and beset with problems. Scientific and technical knowledge is not only gradually destroying both superstition and conventional religion, but it is also depriving many of the faith which sustained their fathers. Unfortunately, it offers nothing in its place, no guiding star for which many people unconsciously long. More and more young people, with highly trained minds, find that the orthodox religious beliefs seem unreasonable and provide no answer to human problems. Such problems have always existed but are now made more complex by the increasing speed and freedom of modern life and the problems facing the planet on all fronts.

Earlier in this book I suggested that it was important to understand that we are eternal, and central to that understanding is the concept of reincarnation. Reincarnation is part of the Ancient Wisdom which has been handed down through the ages. It is almost universally accepted in the eastern religions but orthodox Christianity has firmly denied it since The Council of Constantinople in AD 553. At that time it was agreed, by a majority, that anyone who supported the 'mythical doctrine of pre-existence of the soul and who believed in the soul's return to earth after death' should 'henceforth be anathema'. Thus the church leaders suppressed a truth which had been taught in the mystery schools throughout the ancient world.

In different cultures there are different ideas concerning the nature of the soul's return into physical existence. Some people believe, for instance, that the return is not necessarily in human form but can be in the body of an animal. However, other teachings state that having an individual soul differentiates humans from the animal kingdom. Unlike animals humans have an awakening consciousness of the divine. This progress cannot be reversed and on this basis it is impossible for a human soul to reincarnate in an animal form. The human soul has a free-will choice as to how it will react to people and circumstances. Animals, on the other hand, come under the care and direction of a group spirit who gives them their innate instincts for survival and growth. A group spirit will direct the migration of birds or the habits of each particular species.

The same teaching states that animals eventually attain to the human level of evolution through association with the humans whom they serve. Love between the two can grow, perhaps over a number of lives, till it reaches the point where the animal friend is so full of devotion that it will sacrifice its life for the beloved master or mistress. The growth of love in the animal soul gradually brings such an attachment to the human life that it withdraws from the group and starts on the human path towards individualisation. This surely demonstrates the immense importance of treating animals with love and respect especially those who have reached the stage of their evolution of being drawn to human companionship. Such animals even sacrifice their bodies in the service of their human guardians. This service is part of the great lesson of love which gradually brings the soul, whether animal or human, a deeper understanding. In the human state it seems that the young soul is, at first, drawn into a closely-knit human group, family or tribe. Here, again, it is completely obedient to the leader and to the customs of the group. Gradually, through many lives, the mind develops independence, bringing an urge for individualisation. This leads progressively to the time when instead of blindly following the animal instincts of the body, the soul desires to understand more of the whence, whither and why of existence. Thus, gradually, the soul evolves from the animal to the human and from the human to the divine—to full consciousness of the Creator.

From the beginning of time the group or family consciousness is part of the soul's growth. It seems that souls continue to work through many lives with their family group. This does not necessarily mean the blood family but a group of souls who can work together harmoniously to help one another's evolution. When a soul reincarnates it does so with a certain mission and with a certain lesson to learn. We may find ourselves living and working with those whom we have loved and helped as well as those whom we have injured and hated. The eventual object being to forgive and make good all the hurts, to straighten all the crooked places and to transform all hate or dissension into brotherly love and understanding.

Simply stated reincarnation means the periodic descent of the soul to labour in this world. But creation is governed by the supreme principles of love and wisdom; therefore having lived on earth for a span (which is retrospect seems about as long as the blink of an eye) the soul withdraws from earthly activity to rejoin its true self and to assimilate the lessons it has learned. It returns for refreshment to its true home in the heaven world.

For many, reincarnation answers all the problems concerning the inequality of man's lot in his present life. They are content to know that what they meet in this life, either good or ill, is the result of their past actions. The question often arises about why we cannot remember our past lives. Such memories are stored in the higher self of man and until sufficient spiritual development is attained, or until the soul is ready to face these memories, it is impossible for the brain to receive impressions from that higher memory.

As the soul develops and unfolds, memories of the past start to awaken and it begins to recognise exactly why it is faced with certain conditions in the present life. The soul will accept what is happening, knowing the law is just, perfect and true. The soul also knows that by its reaction to any adversity in its present day life, it will create new opportunities in the future. Many people are already in touch, in some measure, with their past lives which helps them to come to terms with their current difficulties.

CHAPTER 10

Karma—Cause and Effect

The law of cause and effect, known in the East as karma, arises naturally out of reincarnation. Simply put, it means that as we sow today we reap tomorrow. We cannot sow thistles and reap roses. It is the law which rules the countless incarnations of the soul. Perhaps the invention of the computer, with its built-in memory, makes it easier for us to comprehend the precise and inexorable law of karma. Through the supreme justice of the Creator we are re-born always into an environment where we meet again those whom we have wronged or by whom we have been wronged. Equally we meet again those whom we have helped or who have helped us as well as those to whom we are linked by a bond of deep love. This is particularly true of family relationships.

It has long been recognised that the first seven years of life are vital in the formation of character. But, when we understand the truth of reincarnation and karma, we realise that character, although shaped by our parents and the family environment, has been developed through our habitual thought and action in past lives. The soul is drawn to those parents with whom it has some deep emotional link from the past, either positive or negative. The genes of those parents will give the required body and their auras will supply the necessary soul environment for further progress on the path of evolution. In the same way parents draw to themselves souls whose karma is interlinked with their own. They will be able to help those souls as well as learning from them.

Every soul is born under the care and direction of a guardian angel (more about this a little later) who ensures that the individual comes into incarnation at the moment when its first breath enables it to draw in the planetary vibrations which will form the blueprint of that life. As previously stated we learn so much through the experience of our physical body—its strength or weakness, its perfections or imperfections and its health or disharmony.

Karma is the law of cause and effect and following upon this is the law of opportunity. On its long journey the soul receives continual opportunity to attain divine illumination. During every incarnation lessons are presented, tests if you like, which are actually opportunities for progress and initiation.

It is worth remembering that, through many incarnations, a soul will incur certain karmic debts. These karmic debts cannot be paid off until sufficient wisdom and strength has been gained to enable an individual to deal with them. Some spiritual sources teach that no soul returns to earth with a heavier load than it can bear. However, I dare say we have all wondered about that, from time to time, when life has been particularly trying!

Karma must not be thought of as something bad or as a punishment for transgressions of the past. It is more an opportunity to balance the books. Good fortune such as winning a raffle, the premium bonds or a holiday trip, etc. may equally be karmic and a recognition of some kind deed of long ago. On the other hand it may also be a test to see how we cope with responsibility.

So called bad karma is created not only by a lack of love but by absence of wisdom, by ignorance. Until a soul experiences for itself, it cannot know or understand or appreciate what love is. Through experience the soul acquires love and wisdom. However, when we come to the question of ignorance we are sailing in tricky waters. I take the view that man is not so ignorant as not to know that selfishness and greed are wrong, yet he frequently persists in them and in so doing brings suffering upon himself. There seems to me to be a difference between innocent ignorance and wilful ignorance. In the latter case one really knows deep down that there is a denial of that inner voice or conscience.

Karmic debts can be transmuted in various ways. To recognise a past mistake is half the battle. Once aware of an error it is a natural impulse to want to do something to recompense the person one has wronged. If one is aware of having behaved badly in the past then by giving service to the aggrieved person or persons the slate can be wiped clean so far as a particular incident is concerned.

Before coming into incarnation again there is a period of peace and quiescence, the rest and recuperation I mentioned earlier. When we shed our physical body at the end of a particular incarnation the soul sees a picture of its whole journey so far... The decision is then made as to what further experience and growth is needed. That is where the real free-will is manifest. The soul may perhaps choose an easy life or it may be given such a vision of the ultimate perfection that it longs to clear off its debts quickly so that it may become one with that heavenly beauty and peace. In this case it may choose a very difficult incarnation, perhaps with a severely handicapped body or mind, or one in which there is almost unbearable emotional strain and suffering.

Patiently and lovingly borne these sufferings are like a cleansing fire wiping out all debts and leaving the soul filled with love and thankfulness to the Creator. The wisdom and deep compassion gained from such a life will enable it to give special service that will be deeply satisfying. Many souls living in severely handicapped bodies or under harsh and difficult conditions show a sweetness of disposition, patience, kindness and humility which is an inspiration to the apparently more fortunate people around them. By the acceptance of their suffering they create around them an aura of peace and light which helps and inspires all who come into contact with them.

We choose, with a lot of help from more evolved individuals, the circumstances of our earthly incarnations with a view to learning something at a soul level. Those readers interested in reading more on this subject may find the fascinating book called *Life Between Life* by Dr. Whitton and Joe Fisher of particular interest.

CHAPTER 11.

Help from the Higher Realms

There is a plan for all our lives. We are like children who have come back to school and our own soul, although its memory has faded for the time being, subconsciously knows we have come here to gain certain knowledge. Daily life which seems so irksome at times and our bodies which are occasionally so tiresome to maintain are, in reality, the restrictions from which we learn. Overcoming the frustration of daily living is the experience we need to help us unfold the soul qualities which must be developed before we can be free from the bondage of physical life.

Subconsciously most of us long for a better world. There is in some way an attachment to the life of spirit, and rightly so, for it is our true home. Our intuition tells us that we come from a more beautiful place for a purpose and according to a plan. We have come from the world of spirit to live in the flesh where we are imprisoned until we learn to free ourselves.

This does not mean freedom through death because death does not necessarily set us free from bondage. The freedom is best achieved whilst we are here on earth. The release from the limitations of our baser natures and physical cravings has to be achieved by our own efforts. However, having let go of these restrictions, we can, whilst still in our earthly incarnation, enter into the heaven realms of peace, serenity, beauty and joy. This can be achieved in meditation and at other moments of at-one-ment with nature.

On the seemingly interminable journey and long pilgrimage of incarnations you may well ask who can best help us? We are assured that guidance is available, from the higher realms, from both angelic and human sources.

The guardian angel is the messenger sent by the Creator from the heavenly states to help each of us through all our various experiences of life on earth. Your guardian angel never leaves you and is the helper of the soul when, and if, it desires to be helped. Strength and guidance is available on request as it were.

The guardian angel is, of course, present at the time of birth and always cares for that reincarnating soul. We must remember, though that the angelic beings have never experienced human incarnation and are unable to draw very close to man until he learns to control his emotions. Many times does the guardian angel attempt to draw close but it is only in its tranquil moments that the soul is receptive to the ministry of angels. Often we are so concerned with the events around us that we are deaf to the promptings of our guardian angel.

The human guidance comes from a particular teacher or guide, human in origin but now in spirit, who may be attached to us through a number of lives. That guide is aware of the problems of earthly life and understands the sorrows and human weaknesses common to every living soul. The guide also knows that in the course of evolution all will emerge strong and radiant, victorious over the difficulties and conflicts of earthly life.

These discarnate guides, from their higher perspective, see us as radiant souls struggling to learn what we must. Our teacher or guide will have a number of helpers, who come to help us through particularly difficult periods and trials or tribulations of one sort or another. Access to such helpers, with a special knowledge of certain subjects, is possible. An artist might be inspired by a skilled artist now in spirit, a writer, musician or doctor likewise. When a particular skill is being used in this life expertise from discarnate souls with experience in such matters is on tap from the spirit world. Many people get inspiration from such sources quite unconsciously. Sometimes these helpers are also called guides and this is a little confusing. However, we can listen to our true guide, who comes from a different level than the helpers, through the voice of our higher self, or conscience, as it is sometimes called. We must strive to be attuned to this voice from above.

The karma most of us have created in past lives, through our actions and thoughts, has the effect that very few of us enjoy the degree of freewill we might imagine. Our choice is limited, probably by fixations of thought, which are the legacy of our early environment.

In the big events of life such as birth, marriage, work, environment, travel, health, it may seem that we have a conscious decision to make but the reality is different. The choice is very often made, long before, at a deeper level. Our guardian angel who, as discussed earlier, is always with us at these outwardly crucial moments of decision, ensures that we follow the path previously chosen by our higher self before incarnating. Hence the importance of turning inwards, at all times, to attune to the help available.

Our only free will lies in the inner realms of thought and feeling. We have free will to choose how we think and how we react to people and circumstances. Deep within every soul, in the heart centre, there shines a light which is our link with the Creator.

We can choose whether to try to become more aware of that light, that divine self, which urges us to treat others as we would like to be treated. Alternatively we can allow ourselves to be held down by material and selfish considerations until such time that the inner light is practically smothered, covered by layers of selfish desire and thoughtlessness.

Every time the soul consciously chooses to rise in spirit towards the light, the good, the true or the beautiful, the law of opportunity works to create a more harmonious environment for the future. This may take the form of a healthier body and a greater capacity to serve. No matter how difficult our present harvest may be every soul has the opportunity to sow, now, a golden harvest for the future.

Most of us are familiar with the expression that 'everything comes right in the end'. We are assured that it must and does come right so why should we be fearful? There are times in our lives when we appear to have more than our fair share of difficulties but still manage to remain calm and positive; at other times we can be overwhelmed and become very negative. By surrendering to the will of the Creator (going with the flow) we will find things a great deal easier. Assurance is given that we will always receive gentle and loving help from those in the world of light. They are always ready to do something which brings us blessing and compensation if we give them half a chance. So, despite the hard knocks through which we receive our lessons, we will also receive compensation and blessing from the unseen.

We are not forgotten. The help is available but we have to remember that those on the other side can only descend so far. It is all a matter of vibration, harmony and attunement. Earth is of a slow vibration. Mortal man has to quicken his vibration to become attuned. He must raise himself to meet and greet his spirit friends. On the one hand it is all so simple and so clear—and yet, on the other hand, so profound and so difficult to attain. In spirit as on earth, only 'keeping on keeping on' will ensure our progress.

CHAPTER 12.

The Pendulum Swings

Written over the entrance to many an ancient mystery school were the words: 'Man, know thyself and thou shalt know God and the Universe'. This was a succinct way of expressing the ancient principle 'As above, so below, as in heaven, so on earth'.

We can only begin to understand this wonderful principle when we realise that the whole manifested universe is the result of the thought of the Creator. As we are made in this image we all possess deep within our souls a measure of this same creative power. The light, which shines in our hearts, links us with the great sun of our universe and with the spiritual power at the heart of this galaxy. The truth is that man is a creator in the making, a universe in miniature.

Astrologers well know the extraordinary and mysterious linking of people's character and circumstances with the position in the heavens of the sun, moon and planets at the moment of birth. The sacred science of astrology is inherent in all religions. The signs may have different symbols, different names in different cultures but basically they all demonstrate the truth of the soul's evolution from the animal to the human and ultimately to the divine self.

This principal 'as above, so below, as in heaven, so on earth' is also a law of externalisation and thus our inner thoughts and feelings build from the past to the body we have now. That body is our instrument for service at the moment. Those same thoughts and feelings also influence our destiny. The inner thoughts and feelings imprint themselves upon the physical body—as in the lines of the palm, the contours of the head and in every form of the body's expression such as handwriting, posture and gait.

In the innermost self there is a programme showing how our life will unfold and this programme is evident in every part of the body. Particularly observant doctors can usually diagnose, according to physical type and build, the dis-ease to which patients are likely to succumb. A trained seer, who understands how to interpret the signs, would be able to judge quite accurately a soul's character and destiny during the present life.

In the words 'as above, so below, as in heaven, so on earth' we have a key to the study of spiritual science. As we begin to learn more of the full implications this law and the exactitude with which it works, we cannot but wonder at the majesty of divine wisdom and love behind every detail of human life.

There is a law of balance and equilibrium apparent everywhere in nature. It is the law of opposites (yin and yang). The balance between day and night, heat and cold, expansion and contraction, positive and negative currents, acid and alkali and so on. As a pendulum swings one way it must then swing the other way. This law governs every aspect of our lives—of the soul plane as well as in the physical body.

To gain necessary experience the soul needs to incarnate sometimes in a male and sometimes in a female body. However, this change of sex does not necessarily occur in each alternate life. We may have a series of incarnations either in a male or female body in order to gain a thorough experience of the needs and qualities of both or because of some special mission of the soul. Then the pendulum swings back and we start a series of lives in the opposite type of body.

This swinging of the pendulum of life between the two can perhaps give us a greater sympathy and understanding for souls who are at the point of change which can manifest as homosexuality. The change into a different type of body after a run of incarnations in the same sex may make it difficult at first for the individual to be released from the pull of that sex which has been theirs for a number of lives. The fact that many great artists are, or have been, homosexual may indicate a time when the soul, to some extent, lives more in the inner world and can be particularly responsive to angelic inspiration in the arts or sciences.

In the spirit world a woman has opportunity for the maternal expression for which her soul might long, particularly if she had been denied that opportunity in a previous life. Equally, a man can pursue the creative arts for which he may have longed, consciously or subconsciously, over many years.

This fundamental law of balance, which affects both mind and body, acts as a safeguard to the soul ensuring that any kind of extremism can only be carried so far before reaction sets in and pulls us back to normal. This law can cause the personality to swing, in successive incarnations, between introvert and extrovert activity until such time as a perfectly balanced expression is reached.

Any kind of fanaticism in one incarnation could lead to similar fanaticism in the opposite direction in another incarnation. This can be particularly true in questions of religious or racial bigotry. For instance, a puritanical soul, demanding complete simplicity in one life may come back with equal religious fanaticism in the next but, this time, demanding elaborate ceremonial practices. A persecutor of coloured races could well be born in the very race which had been the object of his persecution.

Always we receive as we have given, the swing of the pendulum ensuring that we are drawn into an opposite experience in order to widen our understanding and bring the soul into complete balance. So we learn to reach the heights and plumb the depths of human experience. Gradually we grow in wisdom, tolerance, compassion and humour until we can truly understand the meaning and the joy of the brotherhood of all life.

CHAPTER 13.

Subtle Bodies and Reaching Upwards

As I suggested in the introduction of this book we are not simply a physical body. Beyond the physical are subtle bodies. Linked to the physical is the etheric body, next the astral body and then, finer still, is the mental body. The etheric body merges into the physical as water permeates a sponge. The etheric is closely related to the nervous system. It is this subtle body which registers all pleasurable sensations, and disagreeable ones for that matter! When the etheric is driven out of the physical body by, say, an anaesthetic, the physical body feels no pain. One spiritual source goes on to explain that the etheric also forms a bridge across which communication with the spiritual word is possible. It is divided into two parts—a higher part which merges into the astral body after death and a lower part which is closely related to the physical.

Occasionally, the lower etheric part, so closely related to the physical, is known to linger about its former home, buildings, fields, gardens etc. and, indeed to cling to any place familiar to it, including churchyards. This etheric emanation is sometimes earthbound for a long time although usually it disintegrates with the body. It gives rise to the apparitions known as ghosts. It is not the true self, only a counterpart or semblance or the original. What we call a ghost is the etheric emanation left behind after the death of the body. Ghosts could also be souls, earthbound for some reason or, conversely, a more evolved soul manifesting physically for a particular purpose. These are complicated issues and rather beyond the scope of this book.

The astral body registers the same emotions or feelings which permeate the physical body. It seems that we live a lot of our earthly life in the etheric and astral bodies. Thus we feel pain or pleasure, love or hate, fear and hope—sensations and feelings of all kinds. However we must remember that the physical body is only clothing, an overcoat, and when this is laid aside, man continues to live on in his subtler bodies. Just the same man, inhabiting just these same bodies, with nothing to fear and hardly anything strange to dread in the experience of death.

Beyond the astral planes are the mental planes. These are inhabited by man's mental bodies. I referred to them earlier as being a part of us here and now on earth. The mental plane comes closer to the higher self which is sometimes called the angelic or heavenly body. We are told it is most beautiful in appearance and shining with a great light. Every human being has such a body, at a certain stage of development. It is this higher self which evolves during many, many lives and which, in reality, is the temple of man's spirit.

In such celestial realms dwell the angelic hierarchies, the saints and perfected souls of all ages. Such souls would have passed through great tribulations in this world and, through their experiences in countless incarnations, have evolved and become harmonised with the divine law of love.

As I have indicated earlier we do not have to wait for our demise in order to contact the 'heaven world'.

Many people do it whilst they sleep and are aware of experiencing a real and vivid dream which leaves a deep impression afterwards—a vision, in fact. Such dreams usually come in the early morning, on waking. There are many types of dream and for many of us they are probably too confused and muddled to be of value; and often they are likely to have been caused by bodily discomfort or over indulgence of some kind!

It is possible to prepare for the better type of dream and at the same time develop one's spiritual faculties. However it is not something to be done lightly. One must first aspire to do so from the heart and then, mentally, reach upward to the higher realms. It seems that we on earth must make the effort of reaching halfway, as it were, if we really wish to commune with spirit. As we have been advised earlier the door handle is on this side.

I am sure the elder brethren have a lively sense of humour and love laughter. They encourage happiness and a zest for living but there is a time to be still and that time is when we seek communion with higher worlds. Such co-operation is necessary because the link is a very fine and delicate vibration which works through the etheric body. The etheric body is interlaced with our nervous system and noise or discord breaks the fine contact.

Anybody wishing to make a conscious contact with the spirit realms ought to go about it in a gentle way. Everything should be done harmoniously. Within us is a power or divine will and this can be the motive force which lifts us into the divine realms. According to our soul's awareness it will be taken to the place in the spirit world where it will find both lesson and refreshment and where it will meet up with old acquaintances. Such visions can serve to teach us and stimulate our spirit, reviving memories of the Ancient Wisdom which will assist us in our future work. What has happened in our soul's past moulds its future.

Meditation is the key. The aim of meditation is to bring our baser instincts under the control of our higher self and achieve at-one-ment with the Creator. Thus man, the microcosm, the epitome of the universe, becomes enfolded in the life of the Creator, the Macrocosm, the infinitely great.

There are many ways of meditating but the essence of it is to find the place of absolute stillness and silence within. Thus it is helpful to sit motionless and to do this one must be comfortable. The spine should be erect and held as if suspended from some imaginary thread which at the same time links the meditator with the sun above. Gentle, rhythmic breathing will help us to detach from the earthly self. The natural thing is for the mind to wander and if it does then it is important constantly and gently to bring it back to focus on the breath.

For some people meditation (that conscious at-one-ment with the Creator) can be achieved quite differently. Gardening can be a meditation for some. Writing poetry, listening to music, watching a sunset or simply walking in a beautiful place will make the connection for others.

CHAPTER 14.

Near Death Experience

Carl Jung said the following about death:

> 'What happens after death is so unspeakably glorious that our imagination and feelings do not suffice to form even an approximate conception of it.'

And so death—where is thy sting? Where indeed? There is no sting. I have a video tape called 'Visions of Hope' which is about 'near death experiences'. The film amounts to a series of interviews with about a dozen individuals all of whom have had these experiences. In the various interviews there is a remarkable consensus about what happens when one is considered to be 'dead'. The feeling of peace, light, serenity and love prevails throughout.

One man spoke of his experiences as a child in hospital when his parents were told by the doctor 'he's gone' and whose post mortem arrangements had been put in progress. At that time he was 'outside his body, above it and looking down from the ceiling'. He was attached to his body by 'a blue, silvery cord'. He then experienced 'absolute peace and serenity' and was aware of the 'brightest light ever experienced'. He was also aware of the 'appearance of a being' and he 'looked down and saw a ball turning in space'. He did not want to go back to what he later realised was the earth planet but he was made aware that he ought to do so. As he journeyed back in space he saw the colours of the earth (this was long before the space shots revealed the sort of picture one might expect to see from space) and 'impacted' with it. He went on to make a full recovery and the experience made him realise that there is no such thing as death.

Another person spoke of being very ill in hospital when she was in her 20s, watching her body from above the bed and then experiencing a 'luminous white light with blue in the middle—absolute peace and beauty' and she spoke of 'a light at the end of a tunnel' which she wanted to follow. She was then aware of a presence or voice which posed the question 'Have you really done everything you want to do?' She was also aware of a demarcation line at which point one could go on into the light or be 'sucked back again' to earthly existence. She felt it was not time to give up her earthly responsibilities and woke up to find herself covered with tubes, drips and other paraphernalia associated with hospital intensive care procedures. For her it took away the fear associated with death and enabled her to get on with life in a much more meaningful way.

A woman talked about experiencing a bad attack of influenza. She was unable to swallow and was hospitalised. Later she was unable to speak and barely conscious. Lying in her hospital bed she was aware of going up in 'another dimension' and seeing 'a beautiful landscape, moving columns of light, lovely colours, music, but not in the way we understand it.' The atmosphere of 'love and activity' made it very desirable but again there was an awareness that this was not her time to be there and she spoke of coming back, reluctantly, into her body 'through a dark, damp canal.'

Another man had a near death experience after a severe illness. He had a 'sensation of falling' and 'came to in a place of light and brightness' where he said he 'had never felt so alive.' He recognised some old friends there whom he knew to be dead. He was 'very happy and did not want to leave.' He was 'persuaded' to return and had the unfortunate sensation of 'coming to' on a mortuary shelf where he sat up and said 'Where am I?' Since the mortuary attendant was rather shocked by this experience the 'corpse' felt obliged to get off his shelf and obtain a glass of water for the attendant! After a lot of nursing following the experience of being 'dead' for half an hour, during which time the funeral arrangements had been put in progress, this individual made a full recovery. He went on to say how reluctant he had been to leave 'that wonderful place' and for him 'the best is yet to be.' All fear of death has gone.

Of her near death experience another woman said 'the nearer I got to the light the feeling of love increased.' She would have 'liked to have stayed there'... the 'peace and love was beyond explanation.'

A woman who was in severe pain at the age of 28 was hospitalised and had her head packed in ice in order to relieve the pain. She felt herself 'rising out of the pain like a balloon going up' and was aware of floating up to just below the ceiling. It was very calm and there was an 'incredible feeling of light'. Looking down from her vantage point near the ceiling she saw her body intact on the bed below and also she saw her husband enter the room and lay his body across her tummy, sobbing silently. She became aware of her responsibilities to her children and felt, reluctantly, that she must go back to look after the family. Her new awareness has given her an entirely different view of life.

Dr. Kubler Ross, who has written a great deal on the subject of near death experiences, speaks of 20,000 such cases and has experienced one herself. She was aware of 'light at the end of a tunnel and of such peace and love...' and goes on to say that 'when you come back from such an experience everything is changed.'

If one thinks of the four seasons—spring, summer, autumn and winter and of the continuity of life all around us how can one imagine that human life suddenly becomes extinct at the point of so called death? It is a concept which makes no sense at all.

CHAPTER 15.

A View from the Other Side

Life 'on the other side' is perfectly natural. Normal people with bodies and homes and gardens and all the things they need to lead a perfectly natural, ordinary life. The only thing lacking is a physical body but the etheric, astral and mental bodies, already discussed, are intact. Most people are unaware of these subtle bodies whilst on earth but the more evolved one becomes the more one develops and becomes conscious of these finer vibrations interpenetrating the physical body.

The aspiration to the higher worlds does not just apply to those of us on earth. Once free of our physical bodies (after death) we are not limited to one plane or level of existence. Individuals live at a level that they find restful and congenial but there are higher levels to which they can aspire when they have learned how to find them. As on earth, however, nobody can live on the mountain tops for ever. It is really the quality of the consciousness of the soul which decides where the soul will find itself, either during the sleep state or after shedding the physical body.

Grace Cooke, the medium through whom the following information was transmitted, was born with the gift of second sight. In her early childhood it was easy for her to see the forms and hear the voices of those who had passed on into higher worlds. It happened without effort on her part but in later years she had to learn to tune-in at will to different vibrations or wavelengths above that of the physical. She did, however, always take great care to preserve the balance between the two states of consciousness. If her mind showed signs of becoming too dreamy, and weariness or nervous exhaustion seemed likely, she immediately stopped contact with the other world. At such times she found refreshment and recreation in gardening (very down to earth) or country walks. She believed that being close to nature and the earth was restorative to the nervous system and that it preserved the balance between normal and supernormal life.

The extract which follows on the subject of continuing life is from a book called *Sunrise,* published by The White Eagle Publishing Trust. The words are those of a spiritual being known to his many followers as 'White Eagle', who spoke through Grace Cooke. For those who can accept that such information is available to us it throws an interesting light on life after physical death.

'We are sometimes asked what life in the spirit world is really like. My friends, if you journeyed to another continent and later tried to describe that continent, you would find that words conveyed so little. Moreover, after a while your listener would get tired of your descriptions. The experiences of each newly arrived soul in the beyond are individual according the environment, character and reactions of that soul. Therefore what might bring profound joy to one soul might prove only boredom to another. So we can only answer you in this way, that life in the spirit world is very similar to life here on earth, except that the matter which forms the spirit world is not dense or solid and is more malleable than earth matter; while the spirit world (which is far closer to the physical than we realise) appears as solid to its inhabitants as earth does to man. Nevertheless, all its life and substance has a higher frequency or quicker vibration than this physical world.'

'The first thing a man wakes to after death is a world of his own creation. If he has lived selfishly the people around him will be selfish, for like attracts like. A man who has lived only to worship Mammon or riches will find himself very poor afterwards, in very poverty-stricken surroundings. Having little spiritual substance in himself the man has little with which to build his home. His environment will be a replica of his inner self, himself externalised.'

'The life of a man as he lives it on earth is being transmitted into the spirit life, but with a difference; because over there all that is ugly, crude and distasteful is more apparent, more difficult to disguise and conceal and therefore intensified. So also with the more kindly, affectionate and refined life, which expresses itself in beauty, in art and science and in harmony with man and nature. All these are also intensified, both in the man and his surroundings. Most spirit people are overcome with joy when they see the wondrous beauty of their world revealed, when they see the God-like expressed through nature, art, music, science, healing and in the angelic world. They find they are able to see the 'within' of life instead of only the surface as before. They see this inward life as an expression of all that is good and true and beautiful, an expression of God. We cannot describe the wonder, and above all, the freedom of the spirit world. Spirit people have only to think or wish to be in a certain place and they are there. They have only to create strongly in their minds a garden where exquisite flowers bloom and they are within that garden. They have only to think, to long, hope or dream and their thoughts or dreams become their realities.'

'Life after death offers richer and deeper joy and satisfaction, greater opportunity than life on earth can ever give; because true aspiration brings opportunity to the soul immediately—whereas on earth you may dream and hope, but always seem to be limited by your environment and fate. In spirit man is freed.'

In the book I have referred to 'White Eagle' goes on to explain that if a person truly loves his Creator then he will endeavour to express the highest part of himself in his new surroundings. Thus he finds himself in exactly the conditions to which his soul aspired, with opportunities to study, to work or to research—all such creative joys are open to him.

CHAPTER 16.

The Ongoing Journey

The prospect of soaring off to some sort of vague heaven may not be every reader's idea of fun. They might well be thinking that all they want is to stay here on earth where they are safely tethered and everything is familiar. Their view might be to settle for the happiness they know about. Alas there is no choice! We are all eternal whether we like it or not.

I stated at the beginning of this book that I thought a knowledge of the whence, whither and why could help a person to restore his health and wellbeing and to remove any fear of death. I would like to think that what has gone before will give the reader some food for thought and perhaps encourage him to read more on such matters. I hope, too, that it will give a sense of purpose to anybody who feels there is none.

We must try to live in a serene and tranquil way. This does not mean that we need become too serious or solemn because by doing so we will simply chain ourselves to the heaviness of the earth's atmosphere. We can be very still and quiet and at the same time feel joyful within. We need to look above the confusion of human life, realising that our fellow-travellers on life's road are as confused as we are by the events, emotions and desires which come into our lives. Remembering this will help us to remain equable, tranquil, loving and kind.

In the final analysis the key-note of our lives is

love and service. We have to realise the power of love to transmute sorrow into joy and, darkness into light. Not only should we try to love our fellow man but also the conditions of our lives. We are told nothing happens out of order or by chance and the very conditions we experience in life are those we need for our growth. So let us try to accept with love all that happens and look for the lesson that has to be learnt from the experience.

I have mentioned before that it is important to let go of all resentment and to look upon trying circumstances as an opportunity for progress rather than as misfortune. By taking responsibility for our own situation and by doing so without bitterness we are already on the way to resolving the problems which beset us.

Let us try to open our minds to the warmth and power of the spiritual sun, the life force which comes to humanity to make all things new. This spiritual sun causes the spirit in man to grow until it, too, shines. There need be no separation from spirit where there is the impetus or driving force of divine love.

One of the symbols used in the Greek and Egyptian Mysteries was a great winged disc. Another was the Sphinx, whose wings indicate the power of the soul to fly. In those times there was an awareness that no restrictions could hold down man's spirit, unless self-made. Perhaps we should think of ourselves as having wings on our shoulders? We must learn to fly and, in this way, we can all rise on wings into the higher realms. Before us lies a path of never ending progress. We are all heading in the same direction although our routes may be different.

The ultimate destination may be a long way off but, meanwhile, to use the words of an old Irish proverb:

May the road rise with you,
May the wind ever be at your back,
May the rain fall soft upon your fields,
May the sun always shine warm upon your face,
And may the Lord ever hold you in the hollow of his
  hand.

Recommended Reading

Anonymous. *The Mystery of Healing*. Theosophical Publishing House. 1952.

Anonymous. *Some Unrecognised Factors In Healing.* Theosophical Publishing House. 1958.

Colwin Peter. *The Truth is Veiled*. Synthesis Publishing (Isle of Wight).

Motoyama Hiroshi. *Karma and Reincarnation*. Piatkus Books.

Kubler Ross E. *Living With Death.* 1982.

Randall Neville. *Life After Death.* Corgi. 1975.

Schauss Alexander. *Diet, Crime & Delinquency.* Parker House. 1980.

Schumacher E. *A Guide for the Perplexed.* Jonathon Cape. 1977.

Sellers Josephine. *The Return.* Wessex Aquarian. 1990.

Swain Jasper. *On The Death Of My Son.* Aquarian Press. 1974

White Eagle Publishing Trust. *Spiritual Unfoldment—* Volumes 1,2,3 & 4. 1961, 1969, 1987, 1988.

Whitton & Fisher. *Life Between Life.* Grafton Books. 1986.